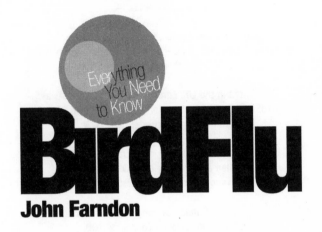

Everything
You Need
to Know

BirdFlu

John Farndon

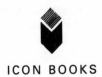

D1413916

ICON BOOKS

Published in the UK in 2005 by Icon Books Ltd,
The Old Dairy, Brook Road, Thriplow,
Cambridge SG8 7RG
email: info@iconbooks.co.uk
www.iconbooks.co.uk

Sold in the UK, Europe, South Africa and Asia
by Faber & Faber Ltd, 3 Queen Square, London WC1N 3AU
or their agents

Distributed in the UK, Europe, South Africa and Asia
by TBS Ltd, Frating Distribution Centre, Colchester Road
Frating Green, Colchester CO7 7DW

This edition published in Australia in 2006
by Allen & Unwin Pty Ltd, PO Box 8500,
83 Alexander Street, Crows Nest, NSW 2065

Distributed in Canada by Penguin Books Canada,
90 Eglinton Avenue East, Suite 700,
Toronto, Ontario M4P 2YE

ISBN 1 84046 749 5

Typesetting by Wayzgoose
Printed and bound in the UK by Bookmarque Ltd

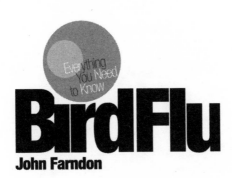

Everything
You Need
to Know

BirdFlu

John Farndon

Contents

John Farndon is the author of many popular reference books on a wide range of topics, including the best-selling Dorling Kindersley *Pocket Encyclopaedia* and the Collins *Children's Encyclopaedia*. He has been short-listed three times for the Aventis Science Book junior prize.

Tony Minson is Professor of Virology and Deputy Vice Chancellor of the University of Cambridge.

Foreword

by Professor Tony Minson

'I've got the flu' must be one of the more common phrases in the English language. Of course, most people who say it probably haven't got influenza at all – they have a bad cold or some other respiratory infection. Nevertheless, it's obvious that the word 'flu' is not one that strikes fear into our hearts, otherwise we would all be demanding a flu vaccination every year. So why are we so worried about bird flu? The answer is that new varieties of influenza appear from time to time, causing world-wide epidemics and killing millions of people, and we are fairly certain that these new varieties, or at least some of their genes, originate in birds.

The appearance of a lethal bird flu that occasionally transmits to – and kills – people is therefore very worrying, but there are a bewildering number of factors involved in understanding the risks and deciding what to do. How does the virus grow, how does it spread, how do our bodies react to it, and how does it cause disease? How does the poultry industry work in different parts of the world and how do the great bird migrations spread the virus around the globe? How much does bird flu have to change in order to become a new human flu? How can we tell whether a new human flu will be a deadly killer, like the 1918 pandemic, or a milder variety like those of 1957 and 1968? How do we design vaccines against flu, and how long does it take to stockpile antiviral drugs and new vaccines?

If scientists, doctors and vets are struggling, it's hardly surprising that the general public is confused. Sooner or later a new human flu pandemic will arrive, and we need to be prepared. John Farndon's book tells us what we need to know, taking us through the issues in a straightforward style and using plain language. His conclusion is right: we are not ready yet, so keep your fingers crossed.

CHAPTER 1

Bird Flu Arrives

'In view of the high mortality of human influenza associated with this strain, the prospect of a worldwide pandemic is frightening.'
Editorial, *The Lancet*, January 2004

On 22 October 2005, a parrot was found dead in quarantine premises somewhere in the UK. The death of a parrot would not normally be big news, but this parrot's demise made all the front pages and topped the TV news instantly. The parrot was, of course, the UK's first confirmed victim of avian influenza type H5N1, or 'bird flu' as it's more popularly known.

Suddenly, bird flu caught everyone's attention. It was no longer something remote, happening to chickens in Asia. It was here, now. People wanted to know just what it was, how you could catch it, how you could treat it if you did catch it, and much more besides. Questions were asked of ministers. Newspapers demanded action. Rumour spread that eating chicken was dangerous, and some supermarkets reported a dramatic plunge in sales of chicken. Wealthy City firms were said to be stocking up on the drug Tamiflu to treat their staff should bird flu make its way into the Square Mile.

For most of us – except for the elderly, the very young and those with chest problems – flu is just one of those annoying things about winter, a bug that lays you low for a few days and makes you feel quite poorly but is ultimately just a nuisance. With the death of this parrot, however, people are finally beginning to take notice of what some experts have been saying for years. Influenza is not just a mild bug; it is actually one of the world's major killer diseases.

Killer flus

Working hand in hand with respiratory diseases such as pneumonia and tuberculosis, certain strains of flu claim a steady toll of hundreds of thousands of lives each year. This is disturbing enough, but flu is a remarkable virus that is constantly changing and evolving. Every now and then, particular killer strains of flu emerge that suddenly sweep out across the world in great worldwide epidemics or 'pandemics'. The most notorious, and deadly, was the Great Influenza in the aftermath of the First World War, which recent estimates think might have killed up to 100 million people. But there have been several more pandemics since, at regular intervals – less severe, but still claiming many lives. These pandemics occur when a particular strain of flu jumps the species barrier from birds or pigs to humans. Human bodies are then faced with a new germ to which they have no natural immunity, and which can prove far more deadly than run-of-the-mill 'winter' flu. Barely 1 or 2 per cent of people who catch these killer flus actually die, but 1 or 2 per cent of the world's population is a lot of people.

The next pandemic?

Most experts believe that it's not a question of 'if' we have another pandemic like the Great Influenza, but 'when'. Many say that the next great pandemic is now actually overdue. At the moment, the H5N1 virus, the strain of flu that killed the parrot, is mainly confined to birds. So far it's known to have killed fewer than a hundred people, and most of these had direct and close contact with chickens. The fear is that the virus may become able to spread between humans. If so, then it could set alight the next great pandemic.

World Health Organization spokesmen are not given to wild overstatement, but in November 2004 the WHO's Shigeru Omi said the death-toll in such a pandemic may be 'in the worst case, 100 million'. One Russian virologist, Dmitri Lvov, says that more than a billion may die. The plain fact is that no one really has a clue just how bad it could be. As the WHO's head, Klaus Stöhr, said in a remarkably honest statement to *The Times*: 'No one knows how many are likely to die in the next influenza pandemic ... The numbers are all over the place.' Yet although we don't know just how bad, the consensus is that the next great flu pandemic will be bad.

At the moment, though, no one knows if the H5N1 bird flu is the germ of the next pandemic, or if it will remain confined to birds alone. Health spokesmen, anxious to avoid panic, have stressed that it's basically a disease of birds, and that we therefore have nothing to fear. As they point out, most of the few people who have so far died are poor farmers who live in very close contact with their chickens. However, in August 2004, a young Thai woman died from bird flu caught from her daughter, who in turn caught it from chickens – and this woman passed it on to her sister, who was treated with Tamiflu and recovered. So there is absolutely no guarantee that bird flu will never pass between humans.

The dead parrot

Although bird flu originated in southeast Asia, the parrot found dead in UK quarantine was actually an Orange-winged Amazon, imported from Surinam in South America, which as yet has no bird flu. It arrived in the UK on 16 September 2005 as part of a consignment of South American tropical birds destined for pet shops around the country. In the normal procedure, it passed through the Heathrow Animal Reception Centre and then went to an approved quarantine centre where it was due to spend 30 days. At the centre, it came into contact with 216 birds from Taiwan, and it is from these birds that the parrot is thought to have caught the flu. Fortunately, it died just a few days before it was due to be released from quarantine, and not after. If it had survived a little longer, it might have left quarantine still infected and so started an outbreak of bird flu in the UK. Naturally, people have been asking questions. How, for instance, did the parrot catch the disease from the Taiwanese birds when regulations say that birds from different continents should be kept apart in quarantine? In the wake of this worrying incident, Britain called for, and got, the European Commission to ban all imports of exotic birds caught in the wild. Some scientists fear, though, that this may mean that the birds are smuggled in instead, and so miss the safety barrier of quarantine. Meanwhile, all 2,000 birds currently in quarantine are being held there until thorough medical checks are done.

CHAPTER 2

Catching Diseases

'... man starts in as a child and lives on diseases to the end as a regular diet.'

Mark Twain

To the hunter-gatherers of the early days of mankind, infectious diseases were probably virtually unknown. These people didn't live close enough together for germs to spread, or stay long enough near water sources to pollute them. Nor did they have the tame animals that today harbour all kinds of germs. But as people colonised the world, so they too were colonised by germs, from parasitic worms to bacteria to viruses. The discovery of farming some 10,000 years ago saved mankind from starvation and provided food for a massive population explosion. But by allowing people and animals to live close together it promoted the conditions which allowed infectious disease to thrive for the first time.

Farm animals shared their germs with humans directly. Cattle gave us tuberculosis and smallpox. Dogs gave us measles. Horses gave us that annoying winter scourge, the common cold. And maybe chickens or pigs gave us flu. As farming became more intensive, manure-polluted water allowed diseases such as polio, cholera, typhoid and hepatitis to thrive, while irrigation water provided ideal conditions for parasites such as those causing bilharzia and schistosomiasis – not to mention malaria.

Humans were by no means defenceless against this rising tide of infectious disease. As each infection struck, so survivors acquired antibody protection, and natural immunity to an increasing number of diseases was passed on from parents to children in the womb or through breast milk.

Waves of disease

But throughout history, waves of epidemics have spread across the globe, becoming increasingly deadly as populations grew and people moved around more and more. In AD 165–180, the Antonine plague killed a quarter of the Roman

Empire's population. About 1300, the Black Death (bubonic plague spread by rat fleas) began its sweep across from the Middle East through Europe and North Africa, culminating in the dreadful years of 1346–50, when 20 million people died and whole villages were wiped out.

Virgin populations, with no natural immunity, proved particularly vulnerable to introduced diseases. When the Spanish conquistador Cortés conquered the Aztecs in 1521, most of the Aztecs fell victim not to Cortés's little band of marauders but to the deadly smallpox they brought with them. The first epidemic to hit the Americas from Europe, though, was probably swine or Spanish flu, brought by the pigs on Columbus's ships. Over 400 years later, another outbreak of swine flu proved to be the worst epidemic ever. In 1918–19, swine flu swept around a world still shell-shocked by the Great War, and killed 60–100 million people – far more than the war itself.

Just as the farming revolution 10,000 years ago brought its share of diseases, so too did the Industrial Revolution 200 years ago. The crowded conditions in the new towns of the 19th century allowed wave after wave of epidemics of cholera to take a deadly toll among the poor who lived so close together in filthy places.

'The English Sweat': Tudor flu?

No one knows just when flu first appeared, but one theory says that it was the illness that struck Henry Tudor's troops after they defeated King Richard III at Bosworth Field in August 1485. The symptoms of the disease included burning thirst, headache, painful joints, sometimes vomiting – and always the terrible high fever which earned the disease the name 'The English Sweat'. The illness was quite brief, killing its victims in just a few hours, or keeping them badly ill for several days before they recovered. After the battle, Henry's victorious troops carried the infection to London with them, leading to an outbreak so severe that his coronation had to be postponed – despite the urgency of sealing Henry's position as divinely anointed king. The epidemic of this mystery illness lasted just a few weeks, then simply stopped. Over the next century, it reappeared four or five times, and in 1528 spread to Germany, where it was known as 'the English Pestilence'.

As later chapters show, increasing urbanisation in the Third World today is repeating this pattern, proving an all-too-rich breeding ground for diseases like flu.

New diseases

New diseases are continuing to appear, including HIV, Ebola, SARS and, of course, new strains of flu. So what we're seeing today isn't necessarily unusual; diseases have emerged continually throughout history, flared up in an epidemic as more and more people came in contact with them, then subsided again as susceptible people died and survivors developed immunity. But better diagnostic techniques are identifying diseases for the first time, and increased global travel is helping spread diseases faster than ever before. The outbreak of the SARS virus in 2003 spread from China to Canada in a matter of days.

An epidemic is an outbreak of disease that attacks many people at the same time. Sometimes an epidemic lasts just a few hours, or a few weeks. But it can last several years. If it stays in a region indefinitely, it is said to be endemic. If it spreads around the world, it is said to be pandemic. In the past, only outbreaks of infectious diseases such as measles and flu were described as epidemic. Now the increasing incidence of non-infectious diseases like cancer and heart disease is often referred to as an epidemic, too.

How you catch diseases

You can catch an infectious disease in a number of ways. Communicable diseases are diseases that spread by direct contact like HIV, colds, hepatitis and, of course, flu. The easiest way to catch one of these diseases is by coming in touch with a person or animal who has the disease.

Touch down

Diseases like these spread mostly by the direct transfer of germs from one person to another. This can happen when someone with the germ kisses someone or exchanges body fluid with someone else. Not surprisingly, then, many diseases are spread by sexual contact – and it's no coincidence that sexually transmitted diseases (STDs) are among the most common of all infections in the USA. Some 3 million Americans catch chlamydia each year, 650,000 have gonorrhea, perhaps 900,000 have HIV, and 45 million have the herpes simplex virus responsible for genital herpes. You can also be infected by hand to hand contact. You often catch cold when your hands carry a virus to your eyes or nose – which is one of the reasons why doctors stress the importance of handwashing. Contact with animals can give you an infection, too. Prairie dogs, for instance, can give you monkeypox, while rabid dogs can give you rabies. Transmission from birds, of course, might prove crucial with bird flu. Unborn babies can catch communicable diseases like HIV and toxoplasmosis through the blood of their mother.

The contact doesn't always need to be direct. You can pick up certain germs lingering on table-tops, door-knobs and taps, especially colds and flu.

Coughs and sneezes

When people cough or sneeze, they blow droplets into the air. If they've got a cold, flu or other similar infection, these droplets contain the germs that made them ill. These droplets travel only about three feet before they drop to the ground. But if you get close enough you can easily breathe the droplets in, and so become infected yourself.

Some kinds of germ can travel through the air on particles so tiny that they hang in the air for some time, and may get blown some distance. Tuberculosis and the SARS virus are like this. This is why these two diseases cause such concern.

Carriers

Some germs are carried by tiny creatures such as insects that come into close contact with humans. Mosquitoes, fleas, lice and ticks all carry disease like this. Some mosquitoes carry malaria, for instance, while fleas carry the plague, and deer ticks carry the Lyme disease germ. Carriers like these are called vectors.

In many parts of the world, dirty drinking water is a major hazard. Human waste can get into drinking water, spreading bacteria, worms and protozoans. Germs like these make diarrhoea one of the most widespread of all diseases. Germs can also spread in contaminated food. Bacteria such as Escherichia coli (E. Coli) can spread in poorly cooked hamburgers. Salmonella can also spread in meat and eggs.

CHAPTER 3

What is a Virus?

'Virus is a Latin word used by doctors to mean "Your guess is as good as mine."'

Anonymous

If you go to the doctor with a bad chest infection or diarrhoea, the chances are you will be given an antibiotic, just in case the culprit germs are bacteria. Often, though, the antibiotic will have no effect, because the germ was, in fact, a virus. Because they often give similar symptoms like this, bacteria and viruses are often lumped together. Yet they couldn't be more different.

Viruses are a form of life like no other. In fact, there are scientists who say that they're not a form of life at all. Indeed, bacteria have more in common with humans than they do with viruses. For a start, both bacteria and humans – and all other living things – have cells, microscopic parcels to contain their life processes. Viruses, uniquely, have no cell. They don't even have the cell structures that living things need to eat, make energy, grow and so on. All they can do that is lifelike is copy themselves. They are actually lifeless, inert chemical particles – as long as they are outside a living cell. Once they get inside a living cell, however, they change completely, taking it over like some demented house guest. Unfortunately for us, they are programmed to do just that.

All viruses have a core of nucleic acid coated with protein, and occasionally an envelope of fat. But this envelope is no more like a bacterium's cell wall than a paper envelope is like a house wall. The size difference is pretty similar, too. Bacteria are, on average, a thousand or more times bigger than viruses. While you can see most bacteria under a powerful light microscope, you need an electron microscope to see viruses. The Dutch microscopist Anton van Leeuwenhoek saw bacteria, or animalcules as he called them, back in the 17th century, but it wasn't until the 1970s that scientists had microscopes powerful enough to see viruses.

Breaking in

The virus's protein coat or fatty envelope is its safe-breaker, and its task is to get the virus into the cell. However, it must be the right cell. The viral coat of each kind of virus needs to match exactly the chemical receptors on its host cell. The cells have these receptors for obtaining the chemicals they need, not for viruses – but if the virus's coat finds a receptor that fits perfectly, it's in.

It's this need for a perfect match that makes viruses far more choosy about who they attack than bacteria. Most viruses live in the cells of a particular species of animal, and often a particular kind of cell within that species. The hepatitis B virus, for instance, targets primarily liver cells.

Once it finds its match, the virus penetrates the cell and begins its work. In an acute viral infection, the virus is not just an uninvited house-guest; it is a pirate. As soon as it enters the cell, it commandeers the cell's own machinery so completely that the cell becomes a virus factory. It's no accident that the term 'virus' has been adopted for computer software infiltrators, for viruses are very much like pirate software, taking over the cell's central processing unit and turning the cell's hardware to its own use.

Other germs

The world is full of billions of microscopic organisms besides viruses, including bacteria, fungi and protozoa. They are in the air, in food, in water, on surfaces such as tables, sinks and wash basins – in fact, just about everywhere. There's even a huge range of these microbes living permanently inside every human body. Most of them are completely harmless, such as the E. Coli bacteria which lives in the intestine. But every now and then damaging microbes get inside your body and make you ill by releasing toxins or interrupting the body's normal activities. Medical science refers to every microbe that is harmful as a pathogen – or a germ in more everyday language. When a colony of pathogens begins to multiply inside your body, you are suffering from an infectious disease.

- *Bacteria* are the germs that cause diseases like cholera, diphtheria, whooping cough, TB and typhoid. They are the smallest living organisms, mostly just a few thousandths of a metre long. There are thousands of species of bacteria, but all of them are basically one of three different shapes: rod-shaped bacilli, ball-shaped cocci, and spiral-shaped. Some bacteria live alone; others cluster in pairs, chains, squares or other groups. They live just about everywhere on Earth. Some can endure searing heat or frigid cold, and others can survive radiation levels lethal to humans. Many bacteria flourish in the mild environment of the human body. Each square centimetre of your skin averages about 100,000 bacteria. Most bacteria are harmless. In fact, barely 1 in 100 actually causes disease. Many that live in your body are actually beneficial, like the Lactobacillus acidopholus bacteria that lives in your intestine, helps digest food and kills off some germs. When disease-causing bacteria enter your body, they multiply rapidly, and as they multiply they make you ill. Some make you ill by releasing chemicals called enzymes that cause inflammation as the body reacts, causing symptoms such as coughs, diarrhoea, sore throats, pains and so on. Other bacteria make you ill by releasing toxins that damage tissues directly. Tetanus bacteria release toxins that cause violent muscle contractions.

• *Fungi*, like moulds, yeasts and mushrooms, are the germs that cause diseases like candiasis (thrush), athlete's foot and ringworm. Most fungi are only mildly pathogenic (disease-causing), and many live in or on your body without causing much harm. Fungi are also a major source of antibiotics such as streptomycin and penicillin. But occasionally they can cause life-threatening diseases like meningitis and the lung disease histoplasmosis.

- *Protozoa* are single-celled organisms like bacteria, but they are much bigger and behave like tiny animals, searching for their own food. Many enter the body and live as parasites as a normal part of their life cycle – living the rest of their lives in food, soil, water or insects. Many live in your body harmlessly, but the plasmodium protozoa carried by mosquitoes causes malaria, and the toxoplasmosis protozoa can be fatal to anyone weakened by cancer or AIDS.

- *Helminths* are larger parasites such as tapeworms and roundworms. When these worms enter your body, they live in the blood, skin, guts, lungs, liver or brain and live off nutrients they find there, draining the body's resources and making you ill.

Taking over

Different viruses do this in different ways, depending on the nucleic acid in their core. Nucleic acid is the programming material of the living world. Deoxyribonucleic acid or DNA is the amazing thread-like molecule curled up inside every living cell. The sequence of chemicals called bases along its enormous length is actually a code for making particular proteins. This code can be the instructions to make an entire new organism – the DNA in every human body cell is a copy of the program for a whole new human being. Or it can be the instructions to carry out the day-to-day tasks the cell needs to perform. Making a whole new organism involves the whole of the DNA molecule, but for day-to-day programming, the cell merely makes copies of appropriate short segments on a simpler form of nucleic acid, called ribonucleic acid, or RNA, or rather messenger RNA (mRNA). That way, the precious DNA is not subjected to everyday wear and tear.

The nucleic acid in viruses can be either DNA or RNA, but never both. DNA viruses, like the herpes virus, make an mRNA copy of themselves using the cell's materials. This viral mRNA then takes over the cell's protein-making machinery to build viruses. RNA viruses like flu and polio can use their own RNA to build viruses directly.

With nearly all life-forms and even most viruses, DNA is always copied to make RNA, never the reverse. But there is one group of viruses that does the opposite. Called retroviruses, they copy their RNA into DNA. It's this DNA copy that is used to make the mRNA that instructs the creation of new viruses. The HIV/AIDS virus is a retrovirus.

So, in essence, once a virus has entered a cell, it takes over its machinery to make countless new viruses. This whole process is very rapid in the case of acute infection. Within a few hours, the infected cell is stuffed full of viral particles, ready to break out and infect others.

Breaking out

Sometimes, the viral particles simply burst out of the cell, destroying it in the process. This is why your nose and throat feel sore during a cold, as destroyed membranes peel off. In other cases, however, the viral particles emerge more gently in a process called budding. In this, the virus leaves wrapped in a bit of the cell's membrane.

While in the process of budding, though, viruses are on the outside of the cell, like flashing beacons telling the immune system that here is an infected cell that must be destroyed for the good of the body. If it escapes destruction, the cell can go on shedding viral particles for ages, as happens in people who are 'carriers' of hepatitis.

The virus can even lie quiet in the cell, not making new viral particles – nor even causing any symptoms in the host. It may flare up every few years like the herpes virus, or not at all. Scientists are now certain that all of us have viruses lurking in at least some of our body cells all the time. There is a theory that viruses may even be major agents in the evolution of species, and that junk DNA (the apparently 'useless' portions of a DNA molecule) are the leftovers from past viral infections which have infiltrated their genetic material into that of the species they infect.

Emerging viruses

In recent years, a whole range of frightening virus diseases have emerged in the tropics, including the Ebola virus, Lassa fever, Dengue, West Nile virus, hantavirus and, worst of all, HIV.

All these viruses are almost certainly not new, but have been brought out of hiding by some change in human activity. The belief is that these viruses are all linked to the destruction of the rainforests. As the trees are cut down, the animals that lived in them are forced to find new homes. As they do, they take with them viruses into close proximity with humans, or animals that are close to humans. It may be that the emergence of deadly flu strains has something in common with these.

CHAPTER 4

How the Body Fights Disease

So, naturalists observe, a flea
Hath smaller fleas that on him prey
And these have smaller fleas to bite 'em;
And so proceed ad infinitum.

Jonathan Swift

When the worst has happened and a colony of pathogens such as viruses or bacteria begins to multiply inside your body, your body immediately begins to fight back. Just how well depends on the nature of the infection and the health and preparedness of your body.

Your body has an array of defences to guard against pathogens, together described as the immune system. First of all there are the gatekeepers – the skin which acts as a barrier to most germs, the mucus layer which covers the inside of more exposed internal surfaces like the lungs, and then the acid bath of the stomach. Even your tears contain a bacteria-killing substance called lysozyme. Harmless bacteria living on the skin and on internal body surfaces help too, by preventing more harmful bacteria getting a foothold.

If a pathogen makes it past these outer defences, it then faces a formidable arsenal of internal weapons. In the blood, for instance, there is a mix of remarkable liquid proteins called complement. Like ketchup on chips, complement attaches itself to bacteria and makes them tastier for the body's phagocyte cells to eat (see below). It can also destroy bacteria by making their cell walls burst open. Then there are proteins called interferons which are released by cells infected by viruses, and which stimulate neighbouring cells to protect themselves. But the main weapons in the body's internal war against invaders are white blood cells and antibodies.

The white army

White blood cells are far more varied and complex than you might think. Indeed, scientists are only just beginning to unravel all their mysteries. First of all there are the phagocytes. 'Phago' comes from the Greek for eating, and it's an apt description. Phagocytes are cells that swallow up germs like minute vacuum cleaners, then digest them with enzymes. There are two kinds: short-lived neutrophils which roam through the blood and longer-lived macrophages which lie in wait in tissues and organs.

What is remarkable about phagocytes is that they can tell which cells are pathogens such as bacteria and which are the body's own cells. It turns out that pathogens have a number of minute features that distinguish them from other cells. Collectively, these are called pathogen-associated molecular patterns or PAMPs, and phagocytes have receptors that allow them to detect PAMPs.

Using PAMPs, phagocytes are very good at dealing with many bacteria and fungi. But they're no good at dealing with bacteria that are coated with capsules or toxins that disguise the PAMPs. Nor are they any help against viruses which stow themselves away inside host cells and so have no PAMPs to give them away.

Antibodies

Antibodies are tiny Y-shaped proteins. There are hundreds of millions of different antibodies, each subtly different in shape, each tailored to lock on to a particular antigen, the chemical identifier on every pathogen. Whenever an antibody finds its matching antigen, its two prongs lock on, leaving its tail sticking out like a flashing beacon. There are five or so different classes of antibody tail, known as immunoglobulins or Igs, and each works in a different way. IgG, for instance, binds complement and phagocytes to the pathogen, ensuring that it's either dissolved or swallowed up. Some antibodies actively interfere with the pathogen's chemistry. Some simply identify it so that it can be targeted by macrophages and killer cells.

Lymphocytes: the Bs and Ts

This is where another group of blood cells, the lymphocytes, come in. There are two main kinds: T-cells and B-cells. While phagocytes are indiscriminate cluster bombs, T-cells and B-cells are heat-seeking missiles, targeting specific pathogens. Together called the adaptive immune system, they are triggered into action by identification markers called antigens that mark out particular invading cells. Remarkably, this part of the immune system has the capacity to learn, which is why it's called adaptive. Once attacked by a pathogen, it remembers the offending antigens and can launch a lightning response if ever attacked by the same pathogen again.

There are over 10 billion of these cells in the body, together weighing as much as the brain. Although they have been renewed again and again, the originals were all made before you were born, ready to fight any infection right from the word go. They spend their lives moving around the body from lymph gland to lymph gland, ready and waiting for the invader they are designed to attack.

The lymph system

The lymph system is your body's sewage system, draining away waste material. All body tissues are continually washed in a watery fluid that comes from the blood. Much of the fluid drains straight back into the blood, but the rest, along with any other crud put out by the cells such as germs and waste chemicals, drains away through the lymphatics, the pipes of the lymphatic system. The lymphatics have no pump like blood, but rely on the continual movement of body muscles to push the fluid along. One-way valves ensure that it only ever flows in one direction. Here and there along the way are the lymphatics' sewage treatment plants, called nodes. Lymph nodes are basically filters that trap germs and other foreign material that has got into the lymph fluid. To deal with the germs, the nodes have armies of lymphocytes, the white blood cells that can neutralise or destroy them. When you have an infection,

the lymph nodes may swell as the lymphocytes multiply to do battle with the
invaders.

T-cells and B-cells work in different ways. T-cells
are the weapons of what is called 'cellular' immunity which directly attack viruses and other
microbes that hide away inside body cells. They
identify infected cells by chemical changes to
their surface. T-cells called killers lock on to these
identified cells and destroy them. Others called
helpers summon the cavalry – B-cells and phagocytes – to do the job.

B-cells are the weapons of what is called the
'humoral' part of the immune system, and use
antibodies to target bacteria. There are millions
of different B-cells in the blood, and each has
antibodies against a certain germ. Normally there
are only a few B-cells with each antibody, but when
a germ is detected, the right B-cell multiplies rapidly within the lymph gland, producing versions
of itself called plasma cells which release floods
of antibodies into the bloodstream to find the
invader. The antibodies attach themselves to the

invading bacteria and mark them for destruction by phagocytes or chemicals. Some B-cells, called memory cells, go on multiplying after the germ has been wiped out — so that if the germ returns, there are antibodies ready for it.

The body is armed from birth with antibodies for germs it has never met. This is called 'innate' immunity. If the body encounters a germ that it has no antibodies for, it quickly makes some — and leaves 'memory' cells ready to be activated, should the same germ invade again. This is called 'acquired' immunity, and is the reason why, for instance, you are unlikely to suffer from severe chicken pox as an adult if you went through it as a child.

Fighting viruses

Viruses like flu are very small, and once they've got into your body, they spend most of their time tucked away out of sight inside cells. So they are very tricky to defend against. All the same, your body has devised strategies for dealing with them.

B-cells attack them as they are moving between cells, locking on to them with antibodies and multiplying rapidly to produce a vast army of antibodies. But if the virus is one that the body hasn't encountered before, this build-up of antibodies is far too slow, and many virus particles have time to sneak inside body cells before the antibody army can muster. Then the fight is largely down to the T-cells.

At first, scientists had no idea how T-cells could tell which body cells were hiding a flu virus. They assumed that the T-cells could identify the culprits only once the virus had multiplied and budded or burst out of the cell. In fact, T-cells are alerted to the stowaway by the cell's own internal chemical transporters, called MHCs. MHCs ferry chemicals from the inside of the cell to the surface. As they pick up their cargo inside the cell, they pick up viral proteins as well as ordinary cell chemicals. So the viral proteins are carried to the surface of the cell and displayed there for all T-cells to latch on to.

Once T-cells identify an infected cell, they deal with it in a variety of ways. T-cells called killers chemically punch holes in the cell and inject a lethal dose of enzymes. This is the only course with flu viruses. Because most flu viruses don't destroy their host cells, the cell itself has to be destroyed. There are other T-cells, called helpers, which work by binding B-cells or phagocytes, or by releasing proteins called cytokines that stimulate them into action. Although helpers are important in some viral infections, with flu the role of the killers is crucial.

There is one more key cell in the fight against viruses: another kind of white blood cell called a natural killer. Some viruses have devised ways to stop MHCs moving to the cell surface and so revealing their presence. So a cell without any MHCs on its surface is likely to be infected with a virus. Natural killers are killer cells that home in on any cell without MHCs and destroy it. They also release interferon, which alerts cells to protect themselves against viruses.

CHAPTER 5

Winter Flu in Action

'A cough is something that you yourself can't help, but everybody else does on purpose just to torment you.'

Ogden Nash, *You Can't Get There From Here*, 1957

No one knows for certain what will happen if bird flu becomes pandemic, but we now have a pretty good picture of what happens to your body when you catch ordinary winter flu.

When you breathe in air containing the flu virus, the virus by no means immediately enters your body. It may get trapped in the layer of slimy mucus that lines your nose and throat, or be swept out by the cilia, the tiny hairs lining the airways that beat 1,000 times a minute to waft away intruders. But if it latches on to one of your body cells, it's taken inside at once. There it invades the cell's nucleus and takes over the cell's manufacturing ability to make clones of itself. Ten thousand new viruses are made by a single invaded cell. These viruses go out to invade new cells and make even more new viruses, and so the infection spreads.

But as each body cell is taken over by an invading virus, it sends out a distress signal as MHCs carry viral proteins to the surface, and this is picked up by the killer T-cells that roam the body looking for trouble. Immediately they see the distress signal, they coat the cell with toxic chemicals, killing it and the virus. Soon the infected spot in your throat is clogged with debris from the dead cells. In rush macrophages to clean up the mess, aided by histamine, which boosts the blood flow to the infected area to get more white blood cells in. Then you become aware of the battle raging in your throat, as the swollen blood vessels press on pain receptors, and the local temperature rises by 3 °C as your body tries to speed up the growth of new throat cells.

Soon chemical signals sent out by the flood of macrophages are generating symptoms all over your body. For a start, your pain threshold is lowered, making your limbs ache. Then a fever com-

Why germs make you ill

Infection by any germ activates the body's immune system, and many of the symptoms that you feel – fever, weakness, sores, pains and aching joints – are often the effects of the immune system's titanic struggle against the invading organisms. Sometimes the infection may be spread throughout the body, like a cold. This is called a systemic infection. Sometimes it can be in just a single spot in the body. This is called a localised infection. Dirt entering a wound, for example, can cause a localised infection.

mences as your whole body temperature rises to help new cells grow to repair the damage. You start to shiver as your muscles contract to generate heat. Blood vessels in your skin constrict to conserve blood in your body's core, making you feel cold and your skin go pale. At the same time, blood vessels in your brain swell, increasing pressure and giving you a headache. Paracetamol or aspirin will reduce the fever and other symptoms

– but reducing the fever slows the body's fight against the virus.

Meanwhile, the virus multiplies so rapidly in your throat that the killer cells can't keep pace, and gradually it begins to spread down into your lungs. Fortunately, the macrophages that have eaten the invaded cells are drifting off through the blood by now, and eventually pass through a lymph node or gland. Once in the lymph node, the viral material that the macrophage is carrying is recognised by lymphocytes that are stored in the gland – and these immediately go into action. T-cells multiply rapidly, swelling the glands until they become very tender.

T-cells rush through the bloodstream to the battlefield in your throat, where the virus is attacking more and more throat cells. Your throat becomes so clogged with debris that you have to cough to get rid of it.

Meanwhile, a single B-cell in the gland recognises the virus material, multiplies and begins to release floods of antibodies – over 2,000 per second. The tiny antibodies spread rapidly through your body fluids to the site of infection. There they lock on to the virus and prevent it cloning itself. At last, the combination of antibodies, T-cells and macrophages begins to take its toll on

A winter killer?

When epidemiologists are trying to find out just how deadly 'ordinary' flu is, they often run up against a problem. Many people killed by flu die because they develop pneumonia. So how can such deaths can be distinguished from other pneumonia deaths? Back in 1847, English Registrar General William Farr realised that in countries where they have a winter, flu peaks at that time. By subtracting the normal year-round death rate for pneumonia from the winter peak, he could tell fairly accurately what was due to flu. This winter excess is still the way that flu deaths are assessed. What this way of calculating does, though, is disguise the massive death rate from flu in the tropics which goes on all year round.

the virus and the battle is won. The important thing now is for the immune system to recognise that the job is done. If T-cells and antibodies go

The symptoms of pandemic flu

No one knows just what the symptoms of pandemic flu might be. They may be similar to winter flu, or they may be completely different. Both the Great Influenza of 1918 and recent instances of bird flu suggest that they could be far more extreme and distressing. Haemorrhaging (bleeding) was one unpleasant symptom. Far worse is ARDS, Acute Respiratory Distress Syndrome, in which the lungs fill up with blood and fluid as the immune system goes into catastrophic overdrive. There may also be a 'cytokine storm' which has a drastic effect on blood vessels, leading to a massive drop in blood pressure – again, as the immune system over-reacts by releasing floods of cytokines. The Great Influenza was also characterised by a distinctive feature called cyanosis, in which the skin turns blue as the blood is starved of oxygen by clogged lungs.

on multiplying, they could overwhelm your body, just like cancer. So the T-cells turn their toxic effects on themselves and the multiplying B-cells. Only a few survive, carrying the memory of the battle with them, ready to fight instantly against any renewed infection.

This is what winter flu is like for most people, but for some it's much worse, and occasionally fatal – notably the very young, the elderly and those with respiratory problems for whom flu can pave the way for pneumonia. For children who are being treated with long-term aspirin, flu can lead to a liver problem called Reye's syndrome, which can plunge the victim into a coma, or prove fatal. Those being treated with long-term steroids or who are undergoing cancer treatment may have such weakened immune systems that they too fall gravely ill and may die. This is why doctors target these people and try to ensure that they are vaccinated against the most likely strain of winter flu to arrive each year.

CHAPTER 6

The Flu Virus

'In essence, it's a destructive form of molecular burglary; flu gets into the building, cracks the safe, takes what it wants; and wrecks the place on its way out.'

Pete Davies, *The Devil's Flu*, 2000

The flu virus is one of the most extraordinary of all viruses. Like a master criminal, it comes in countless different guises. In fact, recent research in southern Asia showed that there may be more than 500 different varieties of flu, and new ones are emerging all the time.

Flu viruses are classified into three broad kinds: A, B and C. B and C have both been human flus for centuries. Type C is the mildest, causing cold-like symptoms. Type B is the one that's to blame for the classic winter flu. Type A is the big danger. It remains essentially a bird virus, but every now and then it acquires the ability to cross into humans, either via pigs or directly. When it does this, people may have so little resistance that a pandemic is a real possibility.

The mutable virus

Although it remains fundamentally the same kind of virus, the flu virus is an RNA virus, which means that it's very unstable and changing all the time. When DNA is copied, it's copied pretty near perfectly. RNA, however, is much less reliable and is copied with a host of misprints. When flu viruses multiply, each individual particle has its own set of misprints. This can create a real problem for immune systems trying to guard against it. The immune system identifies the flu virus by its coat, the antigens that match up with particular antibodies. If the misprint in RNA changes the coat enough, it may become unrecognisable.

This is called antigenic drift, and is why flu comes around again and again. With other viral diseases, like measles, you get it once. Your body builds up antibodies, and then is primed to fight the measles viruses off. So you never get it twice.

Flu is almost the never the same, so the anti-bodies you built up one year fail to identify the new season's style. This is why you can get flu every year – and maybe more often. Every year, as the flu season approaches, medical firms and doctors try to identify the style of virus most likely to strike, and vaccinate the vulnerable against that.

Although the new season's virus is a new style, it's not quite true to say that your body has no immunity to it. Fortunately, it hasn't changed quite enough to be completely unrecognisable. So your body can mount some kind of defence, and eventually defeat it. This is why, for most people, winter flu is a relatively mild illness.

One giant leap ...

However, flu viruses have another trick to play. Every now and then, different flu viruses colonise the same cell. When this happens, their RNA can swap giant sections like people playing happy families. So the viruses can swap traits. If this reshuffling happens to involve the genes that make the virus's coat, this can have dramatic con-sequences, and is called an antigenic shift (as opposed to the milder antigenic drift). A virus

that had the kind of coat suitable only for entering bird cells might in this way suddenly acquire
the genes for a coat to unlock human cells. It
has, in effect, jumped the species barrier in a
single leap. If so, a new pandemic is on the cards.

Until recently, wildfowl got along pretty well
with flu viruses. For maybe millions of years,
ducks and geese have massed each summer on
the northern lakes of Canada and Siberia. As
they drink the lake water, these birds take in flu
viruses. Later, the flu viruses re-emerge into the
lake in the birds' faeces. Unlike human flu viruses
which go for the cells of the human lungs, these
bird flu viruses are happy in the guts of these
birds. It seems to be a harmless kind of arrange-
ment, and scientists have identified dozens of
different strains of flu living in the guts of a single flock of birds.

An uncomfortable relationship

In humans, pigs and other mammals, however,
flu is not nearly so comfortable. Flu in humans
and pigs is probably quite a new disease, arising
no more than five centuries ago as a direct result
of the way humans, pigs and birds became
crowded together in farms and villages. When all

were living far apart, an antigenic shift might have produced countless varieties of flu similar to human flu, but they all would have died instantly without a suitable host. With all living in close proximity, an antigenic shift might readily find a host – and so survive to have offspring.

The problem for the flu virus with this species jump is that humans are not nearly such comfortable homes for them as bird guts. Human viruses usually infect the respiratory tract, not the gut, and so spread less reliably, through the air as aerosols rather than through the mouth and faeces. Moreover, because they are new to humans, these viruses are highly pathogenic – which means they kill their host. This is bad news for the host, but also bad news for the virus, which needs a home. Those it does not kill survive because their immune systems have successfully fought it off. Either way, the virus loses. The result is that the viruses are forced to constantly shift their antigens in an attempt to foil the powerful human immune system.

It used to be thought that bird flu viruses acquired the ability to infect humans through pigs. Pigs' lungs, unusually, can be infected by both human and bird flu viruses. So many of the strains that caused the flu pandemics of the

20th century began when genes were swapped between viruses meeting in pig cells. Indeed, many of the pandemics were actually called swine flu, because they probably started in pigs. Pigs were, if you like, natural blenders. This blending could happen very easily in places like southern China, where peasant farming practices mean that birds, pigs and humans live very close together. Hens are kept in cages above pigs, which feed on their droppings, and pig manure is used, in turn, to fertilise fish ponds where ducks swim. Many flu epidemics were once thought to have started in places like this, including the Great Influenza of 1918–19. But some scientists have questioned if this is actually so. Some researchers have suggested that the Great Influenza actually started on chicken farms in Kansas.

The virus in close-up

Under a very powerful electron microscope you can see that the flu virus is a shapeless envelope. On the virus's fatty coat is what looks like velvety fur. In fact, these are the protein and enzyme spikes that are crucial to the virus's identity. The proteins are called haemagglutinin (HA) and the enzymes neuraminidase (NA). Since the first human flu virus was identified in 1933, scientists have discovered 24 very different varieties of these proteins and enzymes – fifteen HAs and nine NAs. The coat always has one variety of H and one of N. This is because the H is the protein that binds to host cells and invades them. The NA is the virus's escape route. When the virus has multiplied inside the cell, the HA spikes would keep its offspring bound in the cell buds that they create. The NA spikes dissolve the chemicals holding them back. These chemicals are called neuramines, which is why the spikes are called neuraminidase (the suffix 'ase' means an enzyme that dissolves something).

Interestingly, this has recently allowed drug developers to find a small chink in the flu virus's armour. The two drugs that seem to be effective against flu – zanamivir (Relenza) and oseltamivir (Tamiflu) – both work by imitating neuramines and so plugging the virus's escape routes. Because of this they are called neuraminidase inhibitors.

Because they appear on the virus's coat, HA and NA are not just its passports in and out of host cells; they are its identity markers – the antigens to which antibodies react. Each new combination of HAs and NAs that emerges is a new

How a flu virus is built

Under a very powerful microscope, the inside of a flu virus looks like a rather messy pasta salad. There are eight twists of pasta altogether, called ribonucleo-protein complexes, or RNPs. Each RNP is a segment of RNA, the virus's genetic material. Each one codes for a different part of the virus's life. The two that are of most interest are the HA and NA strands, which code for the haemagglu-tinin (H) and neuraminidase (N) spikes on its coat – and so determine its identity and which cells it can invade. It is this division of the virus's genetic material into eight strands which makes it able to swap huge gene segments so easily. When two viruses get together in the same cell, they can simply swap entire RNPs.

antigen, for which the body must develop new antibodies. This is why the major strains of A-type flu viruses are identified by their H(A) and

N(A) combination. Thus the virus to blame for the Great Influenza of 1918 was the H1N1, because it had the first type of HA identified and the first type of NA. The flu pandemic of 1957 was the H2N2. And the bird flu virus that's now causing all the worry is the H5N1. In other words, it has the same type of NA spikes as the Great Influenza of 1918, but different HA spikes. Since the HA spike is what gets the virus into cells, that difference is, at the moment, what's stopping the current bird flu virus from infecting humans directly – but this could change easily with even a small change in the HA's shape, allowing it to lock on to human cells.

CHAPTER 7

The Great Influenza

'A dead man has no substance unless one has seen him dead; a hundred million corpses broadcast through history are no more than a puff of smoke in the imagination.'

Albert Camus, *The Plague*, 1946

In October 2005, American military scientist Jeffery Taubenberger and colleagues made an extraordinary announcement. They had just re-created a living, killing copy of the 1918 'Spanish' flu virus, the germ responsible for the deadliest disease in history. Using a technique called reverse genetics, they used viral DNA taken from a young woman buried in the Alaskan permafrost.

The virus they resurrected now lives in a very secure container at the American Center for

Disease Control, and they are absolutely determined that it should never get out. And so they should be. The germ they recreated was the strain of flu called H1N1. It originated in birds, and under an electron microscope, its haemagglutinin spikes – the passport spikes on its coat – look remarkably similar to the current bird flu virus. But there's one small, and maybe crucial, difference. It has a broader cleft in it, making it more similar to human flu viruses. This is why it was able to infect humans. The conventional wisdom was that it acquired its ability to infect humans in an intermediate step in pigs, which is why after the 1930s the disease became known as swine flu. Some scientists now believe that it was humans who were infected before pigs – which may have more disturbing implications for the current bird flu virus.

However its qualities arose, there's no doubt that the H1N1 of 1918 was the deadliest disease in history. It killed more people in less than a year than the Black Death killed in four years at its height in the 14th century. It killed more people in 24 weeks than AIDS has in 24 years. Conservative estimates say that 20–40 million died, but some experts think the death toll might have been more than 100 million. It was extraordinarily contagious, and perhaps a third of all the world's population caught it. It was also very dangerous, killing 1 in 20 of those that caught it – over eight times the death rate in other flu outbreaks. What is more surprising is that these victims were neither the very old nor the very young but those in the prime of life, the 20- to 40-year-olds.

The Blue Death

Yet perhaps worse than the sheer numbers was the devastating speed with which it spread and the horrific nature of the illness. It was nothing like a winter flu. Victims suffered intense pain and terrible rib-cracking coughing spells, and their skin, their eyes and their ears started to bleed profusely. Worst of all, they turned deep blue as the clogging up of their lungs starved their blood of oxygen – a condition called cyanosis. Very quickly, over the space of a few hours or a few days at best, they literally suffocated as their lungs filled up with fluid and blood, described by doctors as Acute Respiratory Distress Syndrome (ARDS). In scenes oddly reminiscent of the medieval plague, horse-drawn carts drove round the streets of Philadelphia, their drivers crying 'Bring out your dead!' and then carting the corpses off to be rolled into mass graves dug by steam shovels.

Such was the terror that the disease inspired that normal community relationships broke down. Cities turned into ghost towns. People were far too scared to look in on ill neighbours. Some sick people and their young children died of starvation in good neighbourhoods, simply through lack of help. In his terrific book on the pandemic, *The Great Influenza*, John Barry quotes a health official who couldn't get a single volunteer to help: 'Nothing seems to rouse them. Children are starving and still they hold back.' The situation got so bad that some people saw it in cataclysmic terms. The US Surgeon General Victor Vaughan said in October 1918: 'If the epidemic continues its mathematical rate of acceleration, civilisation could easily disappear from the face of the earth within a few weeks.'

The spreading terror

It was called the Spanish flu, or the Spanish Lady, from the mistaken belief that it began in Spain. In fact, it was just that in the air of secrecy in the closing months of the Great War, neutral Spain was the only country prepared to admit that it had victims. Yet nor did it begin on the peasant farms of southern Asia, as some experts long insisted. In fact, it began at Fort Funston in Kansas. There, in March 1918, 200 soldiers came down with the flu, and 50 died. The epidemic popped up in a few pockets across the USA, such as Detroit, where workers at the Ford Motor Company were sent home. But it all died down in a month or so, and health officials forgot about it.

Meanwhile, however, the virus had made its way across the Atlantic. There, troops were still crowded together in filthy conditions in the trenches – conditions absolutely ripe for the spread of flu. By September, the disease had exploded and was spreading around the world like a bushfire. Although attention has focused on the deaths in Europe among the war-weary combatants, Asia was even worse hit. There, the disease encountered people on the verge of famine after a poor summer, crowded together in squalid conditions – just as the monsoon rains arrived. Recent estimates by Niall Johnson and Juergen Mueller suggest that not far short of 20 million people died in India alone, and maybe nearly 10 million in China. No country was worse hit than Iran, though, where perhaps a quarter of the entire population died.

Health officials desperate to stop this flood tide of death tried everything they could. But there was no vaccine, no drug that could halt its progress. Only basic health precautions seemed to have any effect. In America, a massive campaign urged people to wear face masks in public places at all times, and anyone who didn't was socially ostracised. But all that doctors could really do was wait for the terror to burn itself out.

Finally, in spring 1919, after six devastating months, it did just that – then vanished just as suddenly and mysteriously as it had appeared. Essentially, the virus had killed all the hosts whose immune system couldn't fight it off, and it had nowhere left to go. Its offspring, though, found a home in pigs, and every now and then over the last 85 years these pig flu viruses have infected humans to start epidemics and pandemics.

CHAPTER 8

Asian, Hong Kong and Swine Flu

'Better a vaccine without an epidemic than an epidemic without a vaccine.'
Dr Edward Kilbourne, 1976

Slowly, memories of the Great Influenza seemed to fade, and the various strains of the virus stayed hidden away in the bodies of animals such as pigs and birds. People began to feel the flu pandemic was an aberration that could never be repeated.

All the same, when soldiers were crowded into barracks in war yet again in the 1940s, doctors began to worry if the conditions might prove a breeding ground for a new outbreak. In America, an Influenza Commission was set up under Thomas

Francis, and charged with developing a vaccine. With his assistant Jonas Salk, Francis developed the first flu vaccine. What Francis didn't know at the time was that a flu vaccine will work only against the strains that it's made for. The Francis-Salk vaccine was based on the mild strains that had emerged in the 1930s. When an extreme mutation – an antigenic drift rather than shift – in the H1N1 created a new virulent strain in 1947, the vaccine proved totally ineffective. Fortunately, this new variant H1N1 lacked the killing power of its progenitor. Although it infected hundreds of millions of people across the world, only a few died.

From that point it became clear, though, that vaccines for flu had to be tailored to the right strain. Although much less was known about the flu virus than now, it was clear that it mutated so often that vaccine makers had to prepare vaccines based on the latest emerging strains. The WHO set up a research institute at Mill Hill in London, and laboratories around the world began sending flu strains to London for identification.

The Asian and Hong Kong pandemics

All the same, the very mildness of most flu epidemics didn't encourage governments to invest heavily in vaccination programmes. In 1957, a reassortment of haemagglutinin (HA) and neuraminidase (NA) genes – probably in pigs in southeastern China – created a new flu strain called H2N2, which combined both human and bird viruses. It caught most countries without any vaccine protection. Fortunately, this new pandemic, called Asian flu, was not nearly as lethal as the H1N1 of the Great Influenza, producing neither the cyanosis nor the ARDS. Also doctors by now had antibiotics to help fight secondary bacterial infections. All the same, two million people died around the world.

Eleven years later in 1968, a third new pandemic strain of influenza emerged, as new bird HA genes were added to the N2 of 1957, creating the H3N2 virus. This was called the Hong Kong flu, because it was first identified in Hong Kong, but it probably came together on the peasant farms of Guangdong in China. The H3N2 was incredibly contagious, and like the 1957 pandemic spread rapidly west across Asia to Europe – or leapfrogged around the world with airline passengers. Again, fortunately, its effect was relatively mild.

So by the time a fourth pandemic flu virus was said to be emerging in 1976 – again in China – most Westerners were relatively unconcerned. In Europe, after being spotted in pigs, it had little impact, and it isn't thought of as a pandemic. In the USA, swine flu, as it was called, caused the biggest political embarrassment of President Gerald Ford's career.

The swine flu fiasco

On 5 February that year, Private David Lewis, an army recruit at Fort Dix, said he felt tired and weak. The next day, after a five-mile march, he collapsed and died. Four of his fellow soldiers were later hospitalised. Two weeks after his death, health officials announced that the virus that killed him was the H1N1 swine flu virus – apparently indistinguishable from the virus that caused the Great Influenza.

Alarmed public health officials urged action to head off a major pandemic. Convinced it was a vote-winner, President Ford went on television to announce a crash programme 'to inoculate every man, woman and child in the United

States'. Two years earlier the drug company Wyeth had been successfully sued for the terrible side effects of their polio vaccine, and vaccines were never big money-makers for drug companies. So Ford had to pay a premium to get them to make the vaccines. The vaccination programme was plagued by delays and hold-ups, including the drug company Parke-Davis producing several million doses for the wrong strain.

Meanwhile, no one had apparently caught swine flu since the death of Private David Lewis, and the WHO reported no flu deaths anywhere in the world. Still Ford was determined to push the vaccination programme through, and on 1 October 1976, the first swine flu shots were given at the Indiana State Fair. Ten days later, several elderly people who had received the vaccine suddenly died from the rare neurological disorder Guillain-Barré syndrome, and their deaths were linked to the vaccine. As Jimmy Carter defeated Ford in the polls, the vaccination programme was suddenly called to a halt. As for the swine flu, its career seemed to be as finished as the president who had championed the fight against it.

And so it seemed to many as if the days of the flu pandemic were over, and both governments and drug companies lost interest in keeping up vigilance against it. Then in 1997, something disturbing happened in Hong Kong ...

CHAPTER 9

H5N1

'A slight haemagglutinin mutation – a difference of only three amino acids – had apparently allowed the bird virus to open the lock on human cells and infect the child.'

Robert Webster in Mike Davis,
The Monster at the Door

In March 1997, chickens began to start dying on a farm near Hong Kong. Medical scientists called the disease Highly Pathogenic Avian Influenza (HPAI) – in other words, really bad bird flu. It is indeed bad, as Pete Davies describes in his book *The Devil's Flu*: 'It's an ugly business. The virus spreads throughout the bloodstream to infect every tissue and organ; the brain, stomach, lungs, and eyes all leak blood in a body-wide hemorrhage until, from the tips of their combs to

the claws on their feet, the birds literally melt.'
Scientists identified the culprit as the H5N1
virus, a strain that had first been seen as long
ago as 1959. This was the virus that meant
turkeys had to be culled in England in 1991.

The Hong Kong authorities sealed off the
affected farms and killed any sick chickens and
hoped they had dealt with the problem. Then in
May that year, a three-year-old Hong Kong boy
was taken into hospital with flu symptoms. His
symptoms quickly turned horribly worse as he
suffered first from ARDS then Reye's syndrome,
before his liver and kidney gave out and he died,
in under a week. When the virus that killed him
was sent off to the WHO's centres around the
world for tests, no one could work out what it
was at first. Then researchers in Rotterdam
thought they'd try the H5N1 virus, which was
until then thought to be exclusively a bird virus.
It proved a perfect match.

Finding the culprit

No one could imagine how the H5N1 virus had
come to infect a boy. It seemed to go against all
the theories that flu experts had been building
up over the years. It seemed impossible that a

bird virus could infect a human without a dramatic antigenic shift. Yet there was no disputing the facts. Anxious researchers tried to find out how the boy had caught the disease. Yet beyond finding antibodies in a few people who had come into close contact with the boy but were not ill, they could find nothing. No more people fell ill, so it began to seem as if it was just an unlucky freak event.

Then in November and December 1997, two young adults with similar symptoms died from the H5N1 virus. People in Hong Kong began to worry. That December, the H5N1 re-emerged with a vengeance in the city's large chicken population. The authorities at once ordered a cull of all the 1.6 million chickens in the city. It was a grisly task, but it appeared to do the trick. For a while, the flu seemed to have been beaten back.

Bird soup

The following summer, Hong Kong researchers were allowed by the Chinese authorities to undertake research in Guangzhou in southern China, where they were convinced the rogue virus had originated. Guangzhou, the capital of Guangdong, is one of the world's fastest growing urban centres. Already, 40 million people live here in an area smaller than Los Angeles. Soon the whole region may merge to create the biggest urban area the world has ever seen, completely dwarfing Tokyo. With this rapid urbanisation have come all the attendant problems – pollution, overcrowding and ill health. The people need food, and they eat an awful lot of chicken. Guangzhou has a chicken population of truly staggering size, numbering over 700 million. No wonder, then, that scientists fear it may be a breeding ground for flu viruses.

What the Hong Kong researchers found here was an absolutely astonishing variety of flu viruses – over 500 different strains. What was even more disturbing was that they were not only finding water-bird flus in chickens, but chicken flus in water-birds. It had been assumed that pathogenic viruses could leap from water-birds to chickens, but not the other way around. This two-way traffic was confirmed all too starkly in December 2002 when ducks, geese, flamingoes and many other ornamental birds began to die from H5N1 in Hong Kong parks.

The Hong Kong research – combined with other findings revealing an H9N2 bird flu that seemed able to infect humans just like H5N1 –

showed that genes were being swapped around rapidly, and new strains were emerging and jumping the species barrier. As H5N1 began to claim a few more human victims, health experts began to fear that a new and deadly flu pandemic was imminent.

CHAPTER 10

Outbreak in Chickens

'If Thais don't eat Thai chicken, how can we expect others to buy our chicken?'
Governor of Bangkok, advert, February 2004

The conditions in Guangdong make it very easy to assume that bird flu must have started here. However, wild fowl like ducks and geese fly all around the world, and they encounter chickens almost everywhere. In fact, the tremendous rise in the world demand for chicken – which has almost doubled in the last 25 years – has encouraged the kind of farming practice where gigantic chicken populations are concentrated in industrial production systems.

In spring 2002, while flu experts were concentrating their efforts on Hong Kong and southern Asia, tens of millions of chickens caught the

H6N2 virus in California's Central Valley. A large area around a poultry-processing centre at Turlock was the focus of a huge epidemic that spread out over an area that was dubbed the 'Triangle of Doom'. Only no one outside knew about it. As the Institute of Medicine later said in a general report on flu, the Triangle of Doom was hushed up 'by corporate decision-makers who feared that consumer demand would plummet if the public knew they were buying infected meat and eggs'. Other outbreaks followed in Texas, Pennsylvania, New Jersey, British Columbia and various other places.

The following year, while the world was pre-occupied with the SARS virus, chickens in Holland's Gelderland caught the H7N7 virus from waterfowl on nearby canals. It was actually free-range chickens that first picked up the disease, but it spread quickly in the densely packed chicken factories. Pressured from all across Europe, the Dutch government ordered the slaughter of 30 million chickens, a third of all chickens in the Netherlands.

The SARS virus

In February 2003, with reports coming out of China of several deaths from the H5N1 virus, a doctor from Guangzhou arrived in Hong Kong's Metropole Hotel. He was already ill with a virus that he managed to spread to sixteen other guests on the same floor. The infected guests included airline crew. Within days the infection was speeding around the world, with people gravely ill in Toronto, Frankfurt, Hanoi and various other places.

Doctors feared this deadly disease was bird flu, which had finally acquired the ability to spread from human to human. The WHO named it SARS (Severe Acute Respiratory Syndrome) after its symptoms. Whatever it was, it created an atmosphere of fear bordering on panic around the world as more and more cases appeared. The worst thing about it was that hospital staff seemed highly vulnerable to infection.

The WHO began to put pressure on China, where the infection had arisen.

But until the WHO advised against travel to China, the Chinese didn't take action. Then they launched a massive public hygiene campaign in Guangdong, which mobilised an amazing 80 million people to clean streets and houses, and placed every village in quarantine. The campaign, though extreme, seemed to work. The spread of SARS in China seemed to stop. Elsewhere, efforts to contain it gradually succeeded and by June the epidemic had burned itself out. By this time, researchers had found that SARS was *not* a flu virus. Instead it was a coronavirus, one of the viruses that cause the common cold. The virus was eventually traced back to animals in Guangdong such as the masked civet and the ferret badger, which are used for Chinese medicine. Ironically, civets are supposed to ward off flu. Although the crisis was over, the SARS episode gave a frightening taste of what could happen if a lethal variety of bird flu did ever acquire the ability to spread between humans.

Crisis in Thailand

Later in 2003, a similar process set off an even bigger disaster in Thailand and Cambodia, this time involving the dreaded H5N1 virus. These epidemics were costing the poultry industry a fortune, and here it seemed the desire to avoid financial catastrophe may have, as in California, conspired to produce damaging delays. As the *New Scientist* reported on 23 January 2004, 'a combination of official cover-up and questionable farming practices allowed it to turn into the epidemic now under way'. The *New Scientist* believed that the catastrophe started because of a cack-handed clandestine attempt at vaccination of chickens by farmers in southern China. This aided the emergence of a highly virulent version of the H5N1 virus, called genotype Z or GenZ, which then spread either via migrating wildfowl or smuggled poultry to Thailand and Vietnam.

As chickens began to die in Thailand in November 2003, farmers tried to notify the authorities, but got little response. Even more disturbingly, the Centaco chicken-processing factory owned by the giant CP company (who supply Kentucky Fried Chicken throughout Asia) actually stepped up production. In an article in

Le Monde, journalist Isabelle Delforge quotes what workers at the factory later told the *Bangkok Post* newspaper. One said: 'Before November we were processing about 90,000 chickens a day. But from November to 23 January, we had to kill about 130,000 daily.' Another said: 'It was obvious they were ill: their organs were swollen. We didn't know what the disease was, but we understood that the management was rushing to process the chicken before getting any veterinary inspection. We stopped eating it in October.' All these diseased chickens were shipped to overseas markets in huge quantities.

Only after the GenZ epidemic had been raging through the country's chickens for over two months, and two young farm boys had died of the flu, did the Thai government and CP finally admit there was anything wrong. A government spokesman said to the *Guardian*: 'What looks like a cover-up was a misinterpretation of procedures. The most appropriate word is "screw-up".' The EU Health Commissioner David Byrne – who had visited the country only a few days before and been told there was nothing wrong – told the press he 'felt dishonoured'. The EU promptly banned all imports of chicken from Thailand. A mass slaughter of chickens began in Thailand, though interestingly the CP farms were exempt.

By this time, there were outbreaks of bird flu and mass bird slaughters all over southern Asia – in Cambodia, Vietnam, Indonesia, China and Hong Kong. Then the news came of the first human-to-human infection in Thailand.

A great deal of trouble

When we hear that a strain of bird flu 'only' affects chickens, it's terribly easy to forget that they are the livelihood of chicken farmers, from industrial giants like Tyson to poor peasant farmers in southern Asia. When the chickens of a large company are slaughtered in one country, they may have supplies elsewhere in the world to fall back on. But for many farmers the onset of bird flu has been a tragedy. On farms in richer Europe, bird flu can destroy a lifetime's work. For poorer farmers in southern Asia, chickens are their only way of living. These farmers are terrified of losing their livelihood, and are often so desperate to prevent their chickens being declared infected and slaughtered by government decree that they will risk their own and their children's lives to keep an infection secret.

One sad story from Japan illustrates the personal cost to people at all levels. After an outbreak of bird flu in western Japan in March 2004, Hajimu Asada, 67, and his wife Chisako were found hanging from a tree. Mr Asada was chairman of the small poultry company Nosan Asada, and his firm was criticised for waiting a week before reporting the deaths of thousands of chickens. A suicide note said: 'We have caused a great deal of trouble.'

CHAPTER 11

Crisis Time?

'People are upset, but it's better the birds die than we do. We can always grow more.'
Romanian farmer commenting on the slaughter of poultry, October 2005

On Tuesday 28 September 2004, the Thai Ministry of Health confirmed that a young woman who had died a week before was probably the first case of human-to-human transmission of the H5N1 virus. Although 30 or more people had already died from the virus in southern Asia, all of them seemed to have been infected by birds. This was the first sign that the virus can spread between humans.

The young woman was 26-year-old Pranee Thonchan. Pranee came from the village of Ban

Srisomboon, a typical Thai village where chickens were central to the way of life. In August, the chickens started dying of what must have been bird flu. Then, according to different accounts, the villagers, desperate to preserve their livelihood, kept quiet about the outbreak, or slack government officials failed to follow up reports.

Whatever the truth, Pranee's daughter, eleven-year-old Sakuntala Premphasri, caught the virus – either while playing with chickens or helping her family destroy them. She soon became desperately ill, with all the symptoms of viral pneumonia. Pranee, who was working in a garment factory in Bangkok, was summoned home to find her daughter dying. Throughout the night, Pranee cradled her daughter until the morning came and little Sakuntala died. Pranee soon began to feel ill herself, but was assured by health officials that she was just tired. She returned to work in Bangkok, but soon collapsed. On 20 September she died, a week after her daughter. By this time, Pranee's sister was also showing symptoms of the flu. This time the doctors, suspecting bird flu, treated her with Tamiflu, and fortunately the treatment worked.

What did it mean?

Although Pranee was the first victim of human-to-human transmission of the H5N1 virus, health officials were keen to play down the significance of her death. The WHO spokesman in Thailand stressed that Pranee had caught the virus only by 'very close, direct, face-to-face and long contact', adding: 'It doesn't pose a significant health threat, so there is no reason to be panicked.' The point he wanted to emphasise was that this was not a virus that had mutated to become transmissible between humans; it was just a one-off human infection with the bird flu virus.

This is probably true, and there have been few, if any, other cases of human-to-human transmission since. All the same, even if humans weren't directly threatened, it was clear that the repeated infection of birds was becoming a major worry. A week after Pranee died, the UN Food and Agriculture Organization (FAO) and the World Organization of Animal Health (WOAH) issued a joint statement describing the bird flu epidemic in Asia as 'a crisis of global importance'.

More victims

Many health experts also feared that with bird

flu raging through the wild and domestic bird population, it was only a matter of time before it found a way to move between humans as well. Each new human infection sent the medics into a state of high alert, as they searched to find the source of infection. Most of these cases were occurring in Vietnam. In February 2005, for instance, a young Vietnamese man, Nguyen Sy Tuan, was taken gravely ill and rushed to Hanoi's Bach Tai hospital, where tests showed the H5N1 virus. Apparently he had helped his family slaughter a chicken, a Vietnamese new year tradition. A few days later, Sy Tuan's fourteen-year-old sister was bought in to the same hospital, also with the H5N1 virus, and it seemed likely that she had caught it from him. Tamiflu was given to both brother and sister, but it looked as if it was too late for Sy Tuan. Miraculously, though, both recovered. Then a nurse who had been treating them, Nguyen Duc Tinh, also fell ill with the flu – and it seemed likely that he had caught it from Sy. Fortunately, he too recovered.

By the summer of 2005, at least 60 people were known to have died from bird flu – and maybe many more whose cause of death had not been correctly identified. Yet there were no more clear cases of human-to-human transmission.

Nevertheless, the sheer spread of the infection meant that all kinds of animals were being drawn into the maelstrom. In October 2004, for instance, the Thai authorities announced that 23 precious Bengal tigers had died from bird flu at the Sriracha zoo after eating raw chicken. Domestic cats were being infected the same way, and so too were many wild animals.

New strains

What was especially disturbing was that new strains besides GenZ were emerging in Vietnam, which seemed to be the focus of the epidemic. In some cases, too, people seemed to carry the disease without getting sick, while others showed symptoms not before associated with flu, and so were misdiagnosed. In May 2005, the WHO issued a report concluding: 'The pattern of disease appears to have changed in a manner consistent with the possibility that human-to-human transmission has occurred.'

Meanwhile, migrating birds were spreading bird flu around the world. Outbreaks were occurring further and further west across Asia. Finally in October 2005, it reached Europe. On 7 October, fishermen in Romania discovered dead ducks in a village pond on the Danube delta. The discovery coincided with the deaths of local chickens from the disease, which, as one owner described it, seemed to make their heads 'bloat and pop'. Within a few days, more and more birds were found dying all over the delta. The Romanian authorities at once threw a cordon around the delta region and began the slaughter of chickens. Then on 17 October, bird flu was found on a turkey farm in Greece. Poultry exports were immediately stopped – and remain so at the time of writing. But this effort is probably in vain, because it's wild birds that are spreading the flu. A few days later, poultry in Croatia were infected, and then on 25 October, dead wild geese were found in western Germany and tested positive for H5N1. It's highly likely that the disease has already reached British birds.

CHAPTER 12

Pandemic Alert

'It is public health enemy number one. It is the top of our priority list ... the media coverage is not hysteria.'

Sir Liam Donaldson, UK Chief Medical Officer, to the *Observer*, 16 October 2005

At the moment the H5N1 is still a disease of birds. It can jump to a person, but not further. Still fewer than a hundred people have died from the virus, and most have had very, very close contact with infected birds – either direct contact with their body fluids, or through eating them raw. However, there's no doubt that bird flu is having a devastating effect on bird populations, and ravaging the poultry industry. Moreover, most experts agree that with every new outbreak there's an extra chance that it will mutate into a form that can spread between humans.

Just how seriously governments and health officials are taking this threat is becoming increasingly clear. On 1 November 2005, Sir David Nabarro, the UN official in charge of preparing the world for the pandemic, gave evidence to the House of Lords science and technology committee. He is convinced that unless some coordinated plan is put in place, there's a real danger of international communication breaking down completely as governments go into 'lock-down' to keep out the infection. 'Large multinational companies have started to do their own risk assessments and risk planning ... I find them very, very scary. They are about closing down, retrenching, locking the doors, one or two months' survival rations ... their own Tamiflu stocks.' He is convinced that the military will have to take over in the event of a breakout.

Some pandemics are mild, but the symptoms H5N1 has so far shown suggest that if it does become transmissible between humans, it will be ferocious. Estimates of the likely death toll vary wildly. The 1918 flu pandemic killed 2.5 per cent of those infected. So far, H5N1 seems to have killed 50 per cent of those infected. Some argue that this high figure is simply because many who have caught the disease and survived have not been identified as H5N1 victims. Others say this figure is balanced out by many likely deaths not identified as due to H5N1. The consensus guess – and this is entirely a guess – is that maybe 5 per cent of those who catch it will die. Some epidemiologists think that the virus will find people's immune systems so unprepared that one in three people will catch it. This is about 2 billion people. So if 5 per cent of those who are infected die, then the death toll could be 100 million. This is the worst-case figure given by the WHO, but as the head of the WHO Klaus Stöhr says: 'No one knows how many are likely to die in the next human influenza pandemic … The numbers are all over the place.'

It may be, of course, that H5N1 never becomes transmissible between humans. Or if it does, it might be even more harmless than a mild cold. Or it might prove so hard to transmit that even if it's severe, only a few people ever catch it. The answer is no one really knows. But the continuing human deaths in southern Asia, and the raging spread of the virus in birds – with a ferocity never seen before – is putting governments and health experts on a state of high alert.

Our defences against the disease take four

paths: surveillance, containment, vaccines and drug treatments. These are explored in the following chapters.

CHAPTER 13

Keeping Watch

'Any cover up is going to be a true human catastrophe in the event that the virus mutates.'

Alexander Downer, Australian Foreign Minister, 31 October 2005

If it's like other flus, and the H5N1 virus spreads between humans through the air, it will spread very fast and be very hard to contain. Flu also has a short incubation period. People infected by the virus show symptoms and start spreading viral particles in just two days – unlike SARS which takes up to ten days to become infectious. Computer models show how the flu could spread, and health experts have calculated that to contain an outbreak, they have to catch it completely within 30 days of the very first infection.

After 30 days, they believe, it will be out of the box and little can be done to stop it spreading right around the world.

Thirty days is much shorter than you might think. A flu victim might catch the virus, fall ill and go to her doctor a few days later. The local doctor doesn't immediately suspect bird flu and a few more days are lost. Finally a doctor decides to test for bird flu. He sends off samples to be tested. The test results take a few more days to come through. Finally, the doctor contacts the health department to notify them. A few more days are lost here. Eventually, the WHO are called in, and devise a plan to contain the outbreak – but by that time the 30 days are almost up.

Surveillance

This scenario is the reason why the various world health organisations such as the WHO are trying to monitor outbreaks all around the world continually. Every time news of an outbreak occurs, researchers move in and analyse the virus strain and assess its ability to spread. The next pandemic could start anywhere, but most experts think it's likely to start in southern Asia. Bird flu has already gained a powerful hold there, and poor people live very close to the birds. Unfortunately, despite the best efforts of the governments, surveillance is patchy. These are mostly poor countries – especially Vietnam – and often the low level, or lack, of support from richer countries has allowed them to struggle too much by themselves.

Containment

If an outbreak does occur, tracing contacts and isolating them would probably not be enough to halt the spread of the disease. But recent research suggests that containment measures would work if combined with partial vaccination and a massive input of antiviral drugs like Tamiflu.

Because no one knows what the exact strain of flu is until it appears, it's impossible to prepare a perfect vaccine in advance of the first outbreak. However, some experts believe a vaccine based on the existing GenZ H5N1 strains could at least give partial protection. One scientist has calculated that this would make someone 30 per cent less likely to be infected. This isn't much, but it might just buy a little time for other containment measures to take effect.

As the next chapter makes clear, there's no way Western governments are going to have time to vaccinate everyone against the right flu strain after it emerges as a pandemic. So some people argue that it makes much more sense for the world to put vaccination and antiviral drug resources into flu hotspots, to contain any outbreak and keep it local. This is such an unusual way of thinking that it seems at the moment to be beyond Western governments. At present, the Vietnamese government is pleading desperately with richer nations for help building up a stockpile of antiviral drugs. At the moment the Vietnamese government has enough drugs for 60,000 people. To contain an outbreak, Vietnamese officials feel they will need 50 times as much, and they simply cannot afford it – especially in the wake of the crisis that has seen the slaughter of tens of millions of chickens in Vietnam.

If the pandemic does break out and go global, experts expect it will run around the world in two or three waves. Each wave may last several months, and they may be up to four months apart. But they will peak locally about five weeks after they arrive.

Local measures

Each country has begun to work out its own strategy for dealing with the pandemic once it arrives. Rich countries might consider giving people antiviral drugs to stop the spread of infection. Certainly, major companies are suggesting they might do this for their employees. However, no country has even remotely enough of these drugs to protect a significant proportion of its people for long. The drugs wear off within less than a month. So if the flu doesn't arrive exactly when predicted, the drugs will be wasted – even on those lucky enough to get them. This is why, in July 2005, the British government announced that it would be using its stockpile of antiviral drugs only for treating those who are actually ill, rather than protecting the well.

As the following chapter shows, there are problems with vaccination, too. So essentially, the health authorities in the UK and other countries are going to have to fall back on conventional measures to slow the spread of disease. As the NHS says:

Since vaccines and antiviral drugs are likely to be in limited supply, especially at the onset of a pandemic, other public health and 'social' interventions may be the only available countermeasures to slow the spread of the disease. Measures such as hand washing, and limiting non-essential travel and mass gatherings of people may slow the spread of the virus to reduce the impact and 'buy' valuable time.

CHAPTER 14

What About Vaccines?

'Final decisions [on who will receive vaccinations] *will be based on advice from the JCVI and the UK National Influenza Pandemic Committee.'*

National Health Service, *Pandemic Flu: Frequently Asked Questions*

Vaccines are one of the best lines of defence in any epidemic. By exposing you to dead or harmless versions of pathogens, they prime your body's immune system to fight future attacks, by generating antibodies and white blood cells. Many once major diseases such as diphtheria, polio, measles and whooping cough are now quite rare thanks to mass vaccination or immunisation. Smallpox, for instance, although once widespread, has been almost wiped out.

There's no doubt that if a vaccine were available against pandemic flu long enough in advance, it would be by far the most reliable way of protecting people and preventing the spread of the disease. Annually administered flu jabs have proved very valuable in reducing the dangers of ordinary winter flu. These work because winter flu spreads only slowly. So researchers have time to work out in the spring each year which are the three emerging strains most likely to cause problems later in the year.

The appropriate strains are then supplied to the pharmaceutical companies who use reverse genetics to make a seed virus for each. They then inject the seed virus into fertilised eggs laid by hens in hygienic conditions. The viruses then multiply inside the eggs to provide a supply that is chemically treated to leave just the antigens to be injected and stimulate the immune system. The whole process takes about six months, and there's no real way of shortening it. Some companies are experimenting with cell cultures rather than eggs to speed up the production process, but pharmaceutical companies don't have enough incentive to invest in this new technology.

All this works quite well for the winter flu, because researchers can predict with some confidence which strains are likely to be prevalent in the coming winter. So the patient's immune system is stimulated to create antibodies that match exactly the flu pathogens, giving maximum protection. Even with the best match, no influenza vaccine prevents illness entirely, but they certainly reduce the chances of the illness becoming serious.

The problem with pandemic flu is that no one knows just which strain of flu is going to emerge as the killer – until it emerges. Once it reveals itself, the first wave of infection is likely to spread across the world so quickly that there's no chance to get a vaccine out in time. It will take four months at a minimum to get a vaccine ready, and it's more likely to take eight months. So it's highly unlikely that anyone can be vaccinated against the first wave of infection.

A vaccine could be ready for the second wave, but there's a limit to how much vaccine pharmaceutical companies can make in time. These companies have found that there's never as much money to be made out of vaccines as there is out of drugs, so their production capacity isn't that big. Around the world, barely 300 million doses of flu vaccine are made each year, mostly in Europe, and 95 per cent of it goes to Europe and

North America. Even if all that capacity were turned over to making vaccines against pandemic flu, it would be enough to protect only 150 million people around the world, since two doses are needed. Moreover, it's not at all clear that the companies should stop producing the annual vaccine against winter flu in order to switch over to the pandemic vaccine.

In view of this, the British government decided to take a gamble in July 2005 and start stockpiling a vaccine against the H5N1 virus. There's a chance that the killer might turn out to be some completely different strain and the vaccine will be totally useless. However, health experts decided that there's a reasonable chance it will be an H5N1 strain. The vaccine will not provide total protection, of course, since it won't be a good match, but it could reduce the severity of the illness and prevent a few deaths. The government has ordered enough of the vaccine to inoculate 1 million people. Even the first doses will not be ready until spring 2006.

The NHS admits there will be enough vaccine only for a select few. It says: 'Healthcare workers and other essential service key workers will need to take precedence over other groups, as it will be important to maintain health and other essential services. Those groups most at risk of serious illness will then receive the vaccine as supplies increase.' Apparently the decision as to who will get a jab and who won't is down to an independent government advisory committee called the Joint Committee on Vaccination and Immunisation (JCVI).

CHAPTER 15

What About Drugs?

'We've seen recently some very large purchases at the wholesale level, companies or large entities who are hoarding Tamiflu right now.'
US spokesman for Roche speaking about the decision to halt shipments to private sector clients in the USA

With little prospect of a timely rescue with vaccines, health experts are pinning their hopes on antiviral drugs. Antivirals are drugs that are effective against viruses.

The most widely used flu drug is amantadine, sold under the brand name Symmetrel. This has been used to treat severe cases of A-type flu since the 1970s. It works by interfering with the viral protein that 'undresses' the virus ready for action once it has got into a cell.

In Western countries, amantadine is used only to treat human flu. In China, however, farmers desperate to treat their sick chickens – or prevent them getting sick – are thought to have given them huge doses of amantadine, with the approval of the Chinese Agriculture Ministry. This broke international livestock breeding agreements. An estimated 2.6 billion doses of amantadine have been given to Chinese chickens.

Most experts believe this is why this drug has now become totally useless against the H5N1 virus, as resistant strains have evolved. 'It's definitely an issue if there's a pandemic. Amantadine is off the table', said Richard Webby, an influenza expert at St Jude Children's Research Hospital in Memphis. Health experts believe the loss of this drug was a real blow, because it was cheap and widely available.

Now there are only two antivirals that can be used to treat the pandemic flu – oseltamivir and zanamivir. Oseltamivir is marketed as Tamiflu by Roche and zanamivir is marketed as Relenza by GlaxoSmithKlein. Both work in a different way from amantadine. Instead of interfering with the virus as it breaks into a cell, they interfere as it tries to get out. To break out of the cell, the viruses have to dissolve the neuramines, the chemicals that drew them into the cell. They do this with an enzyme in their coats called neuraminidase. Tamiflu and Relenza work by replacing the neuramine with a very similar chemical and so prevent the virus escaping. This is why they are called neuraminidase inhibitors.

Although flu viruses in Japan have been found to resist Tamiflu, so far these have been only weak strains. Most experts think that because of the way the drugs work, Tamiflu and Relenza are unlikely to encounter serious resistance. Others are not so sure. Researchers in Tokyo warn that 'further investigation is necessary to determine the prevalence of oseltamivir-resistant H5N1 viruses among patients treated with this drug'. At present, though, Tamiflu and Relenza are the world's only initial defence against a flu pandemic.

Of the two, Tamiflu is by far the more popular because it can be taken as a course of eight to twelve tablets over a week. Relenza has to be inhaled. The problem with Tamiflu, though, is that there just isn't enough of it. Indeed, there's already a mad scramble to hoard what little there is. The WHO urged Western governments to pool their Tamiflu stocks to send to southeast Asia to try to contain the spread of flu. But as Jocelyn Kaiser in *Science* magazine puts it: 'Whether countries will voluntarily ship their own precious stockpiles overseas to fight a faraway plague remains to be seen.' The British government has ordered a stockpile of 15 million doses, but they are all for use in the UK.

In mid-October 2005, American and European governments negotiated with Roche, the Swiss pharmaceuticals giant, a billion pounds' worth of contracts to produce Tamiflu as fast as they could. However, Roche's production capacity is tiny compared to the demand. At present, they are able to make only about 10 million doses a year – a tiny fraction of what the world will need if a pandemic begins. Late in October, Roche came under huge pressure to license the drug out to other companies to make. For a while they resisted, arguing that the production process was too complex. Finally they relented, and Indian pharmaceutical company Cipra and others are now licensed to make Tamiflu as well.

Whatever the outcome of the pandemic scare, there's no doubt that Roche have done extremely well out of it. On 20 October 2005, shares in the company reached a record high and it announced that sales for the previous three months were up £4 billion on the same period in 2004.

It must have been almost with glee that

William Burns, head of pharmaceuticals at Roche, commented: 'Following four ducks in Romania carrying avian flu, Europe has gone mad. I don't think it's possible to find a single packet of Tamiflu in Paris any more.' Tamiflu is now available over the internet, and prices are escalating – especially in Italy and France, but even in the UK.

It will be interesting to see how desperately people cling on to their own personal stock if a pandemic does break out – or if the pandemic never happens, how many individuals, companies and governments will come to rue spending so much money. At present there's no knowing just when a pandemic will start – or even if it will. In this age of science, we like everything to be at least predictable, if not controllable. Sadly, nature always has its ways of catching us by surprise.

It seems highly likely that bird flu will continue to spread among wild birds and poultry. For them, bird flu is already a pandemic. But there's no way of knowing if this virus, or any other flu virus, will ever become able to spread between humans to the same degree as in earlier flu pandemics. There are certainly enough danger signals to suggest that this might happen, and might happen soon. But there's no certainty that it will. Nor is there any certainty that any of the measures taken by governments, scientists, health officials and even ordinary people will stem the killing tide if it begins – nor any certainty that they won't.

All we can say is that governments around the world consider the risk substantial enough to spend many billions of pounds on drugs and vaccines and preparing emergency plans to combat the pandemic. If the pandemic never comes, or is very mild, or if the defence measures put in place prove misguided, then all this money will have been totally wasted. Only the big pharmacy companies will have benefited. On the other hand, they might just save humanity.

CHAPTER 16

What Can I Do if the Bird Flu Comes?

Who will get the pandemic flu?

The short answer is that no one knows. While the elderly, the young and those with respiratory problems are at risk with winter flu, the fittest young adults seem to be cut down by the H5N1 virus – as they were in the 1918 pandemic. The very vigour of a person's immune system as it goes into action can destroy the lungs. But until the strain actually emerges, no one knows who will prove most vulnerable. We can't even tell what proportion of people will be affected, though experts are guessing that up to 1 in 3 could be infected and 1 in 60 may die.

What are the symptoms?

The symptoms could be similar to a severe flu – with a sudden fever, aching muscles, headache, extreme tiredness, a cough and a sore throat. But conjunctivitis has been present in most minor cases of human bird flu so far. And in serious cases, victims have suffered bleeding and acute respiratory problems as the body's immune system fights back, clogging the lungs with blood and fluid. Diarrhoea and vomiting have also occurred. If a pandemic starts, though, no one can tell what the symptoms will be, since they depend on the nature of the strain. In previous strains it was extreme respiratory problems and liver damage that killed people.

What can I do to avoid it?

It seems pretty likely that the virus will spread as winter flu does, through the air when people cough and sneeze. So there are basic measures you can take to reduce your chances of catching – and spreading – the disease. Despite the sudden availability of face masks on the internet, these are unlikely to prove much use. The measures below seem trivial but are still worth taking.

- Cover your mouth and nose when coughing and sneezing
- Dispose of used tissues and handkerchiefs promptly
- Avoid crowded places and non-essential travel
- Above all, be as hygienic as you can – wash your hands frequently, using soap and water
- Wipe clean door-handles, kitchen work surfaces and other hard surfaces that people touch regularly

Should I have a flu jab?

If you are one of the people at higher risk from winter flu, you should have your normal jab. It won't protect you against pandemic flu, but it will protect you against winter flu, which won't disappear simply because there is competition. The government will decide who they want to vaccinate against pandemic flu.

Should I buy Tamiflu?

This an entirely personal decision, but there are very strong arguments against buying the drug. There is a world shortage of Tamiflu now, for instance, and the more that is hoarded, the less there is for those who really need it. Moreover, careless use of the drug may help build up resistance to it, with disastrous consequences for all. Also Tamiflu has a limited shelf life, so could well be useless by the time you need it. Nor will you know yourself when you do actually need to take it. Worse still, you could expose yourself to unwanted side effects. On the other hand, it may be your only way to survive in a pandemic.

Is it safe to eat chicken?

At present, many countries like the UK have banned the import of chicken from countries affected by bird flu. Bird flu has not yet been discovered in British chickens, so they should be completely safe to eat. However, it may arrive soon. It's always dangerous to eat raw chicken, but now it makes sense to take extra care. Eating cooked chicken is safe – even if imported from an affected country – since proper cooking kills any virus. Heat over 70°C kills the virus in half an hour; heat over 80°C kills the virus in just a minute. However, all uncooked chicken meat, including frozen meat, should be handled hygienically. Wash your hands after contact with raw meat and keep raw meat separate from other foods. Cut the meat only on a washable surface, and wash this thoroughly after use.

Is it safe to eat eggs?

Yes, especially British eggs. But they should be cooked properly. If you're making dishes such as mayonnaise and mousse, it's worth checking that the eggs come from a reputable source. Also, bird faeces can contaminate eggshells. All eggs should be washed before they are sold, but it's well worth taking extra care; you should wash the outside of the eggs, and also wash your hands after handling them.

I am thinking of travelling to Asia. How should I protect myself against bird flu?

The risk for travellers to countries like Vietnam and Thailand where bird flu is widespread is still considered low. However, you should avoid places where you or other people have close contact with farms or live bird markets. Make sure all uncooked poultry and eggs are handled hygienically. Always cook them well before eating. If you're staying in an affected area near farms for some time, especially in Vietnam, it's probably worth asking your doctor for an antiviral drug such as Tamiflu, since it might be hard to get if an outbreak starts. Always follow the doctor's advice on using the drug.

How does bird flu spread to humans?

At the moment, it seems that only people in very close contact with infected birds or poultry can catch bird flu. The virus is then transmitted in bird faeces or respiratory secretions. There have only been a few cases of human-to-human transmission. In a pandemic, though, it would probably spread as an aerosol – through coughs and sneezes, through mutual touching of surfaces, and the exchange of bodily fluids.

What should I do if I think I have bird flu?

At the moment, many people get respiratory infections, colds and winter flu every day, and the chance that your symptoms are bird flu is extremely low. If you have just returned from Asia and you are experiencing any of the symptoms outlined above, you should seek medical advice, telling them about your trip, including any visits you made to farms or markets in Asia. Otherwise, go to your doctor as you normally would. Should a pandemic begin, health officials will announce what people should do.

Will antibiotics work?

No. Pandemic flu is a virus, and antibiotics work only against bacteria. However, if you develop pneumonia as a result of the flu, your doctor may give you antibiotics.

How likely is it to happen?

The 64-million-dollar question. Governments have got egg on their faces in the past by suggesting a major pandemic was on its way, only to be proved embarrassingly wrong – as happened to the US government over swine flu in 1976. The truth is that no one has any way of knowing. A pandemic flu might break out tomorrow – or it might never happen. All we can say is that more experts than usual concur that a pandemic is likely some time in the near future, but can't tell how severe it will be. We'll have to keep our fingers crossed ...

50 Facts that Should Change the World

Jessica Williams

- A third of the world is at war
- Cars kill two people every minute
- America spends more on pornography than it does on foreign aid
- More than 150 countries use torture

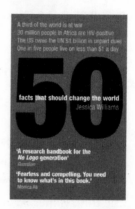

Think you know what's going on in the world?

Jessica Williams will make you think again.

Read about hunger, poverty, human rights abuses, unimaginable wealth, the drugs trade, corruption, gun culture, the abuse of our environment and much more in this shocking bestseller.

'A research handbook for the *No Logo* generation'
Guardian
'Fearless and compelling. You need to know what's in this book.' Monica Ali

How to Give to Charity

Jessica Williams

Charity is headline
news. But with so
many charities, and
innumerable good
causes, where should
your money go?

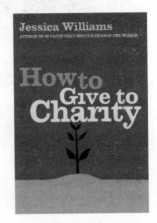

How can you know
that your donation is
being used effectively?
Which are the biggest
and best charities?
Is giving money all you can do?

Is charity the best way to alleviate poverty, cure
disease, save the environment or support the arts?
Doesn't it just relieve our guilt over the world's
inequalities? How much do other people give?

Jessica Williams' new book unravels what modern
charity is all about. It's the essential read for
anyone wanting to help others less fortunate than
themselves.

howtogivetocharity.org

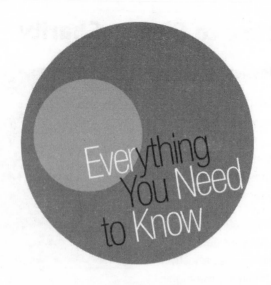

Arresting books providing essential background to topics making the news.

Everything You Need to Know is a brand-new occasional series from **Icon Books**. Produced very quickly in reaction to world events, each book will delve beneath the headlines to give you the crucial facts and real debates behind the stories of the moment.

For more information, visit:
iconbooks.co.uk/everything